SHIBARI FOR BEGINNERS

Everything you want to know about Kinbaku and Japanese Rope Bondage for Safe and Sensual Shibari

Francis McLanahan

Table of Contents

CHAPTER ONE
What is Shibari?

Shibari, also known as Kinbaku, is a form of Japanese bondage that involves the intricate and artistic tying of a person using ropes. The term "Shibari" means "to tie" in Japanese, while "Kinbaku" translates to "tight binding." It is not merely a method of restraint; rather, it is considered a form of erotic and aesthetic expression.

A Brief History of Shibari

Shibari has its roots in the ancient Japanese martial art of hojojutsu, which involved restraining prisoners using cord. Over time, these techniques evolved into a more sensual and artistic form of bondage. The Edo period (1603-1868) saw the emergence of kabuki theater, where rope tying was used as a method of restraint and punishment in dramatic performances. This laid the foundation for the later development of Shibari as an art form.

In the 20th century, artists and photographers like Itoh Seiu and Nobuyoshi Araki played pivotal roles in popularizing Shibari as a distinct form of erotic expression. Today, Shibari has transcended its historical roots and is practiced worldwide as a consensual and artistic activity.

The Cultural Significance of Shibari:

Shibari goes beyond mere restraint; it is often considered a form of communication and connection between partners. The intricate patterns created by the ropes emphasize both the vulnerability and beauty of the person being tied. In Japanese culture, there is an appreciation for the aesthetic aspects of rope bondage, and it is often viewed as a performance art.

Why Practice Shibari?

People engage in Shibari for various reasons, including:

Intimacy and Connection: Shibari can enhance the emotional and physical connection between partners. The process of tying and being tied fosters trust, communication, and intimacy.

Aesthetic Expression: Many practitioners appreciate Shibari for its artistic and visually stunning qualities. The patterns and designs created with the ropes are often considered beautiful and intricate.

Sensory Exploration: The sensation of the ropes against the skin, combined with the physical restriction, can provide a unique and heightened sensory experience.

Erotic Pleasure: Shibari is often incorporated into BDSM practices and can contribute to the exploration of power dynamics and sexual pleasure within a consensual context.

Catharsis and Mindfulness: Some practitioners find Shibari to be a meditative and therapeutic activity. The process of tying and being tied can be a way to achieve a state of mindfulness and relaxation.

Rope: Choose ropes made of natural fibers like jute or hemp, as they are soft, have a bit of grip, and are less likely to cause friction burns. The length and thickness of the rope depend on personal preference and the type of ties you want to create.

Safety Shears: Have safety shears or medical scissors on hand to quickly cut the ropes in case of an emergency.

Safety Gear: Consider using safety gear like blindfolds, gags, or harnesses if part of your Shibari practice involves them.

Mat or Cushion: Use a comfortable surface for the person being tied to sit or lie on during the session.

Safety and Consent:

Communication: Establish clear communication with your partner before starting a Shibari session. Discuss boundaries, preferences, and any health concerns.

Consent: Obtain explicit consent for each tie and any additional activities involved in the session. Ensure that both partners feel comfortable and are aware of their roles and responsibilities.

Emergency Plan: Have a plan in case something goes wrong. Keep safety shears accessible and know how to quickly release the person being tied.

Basic Knots and Techniques

Single and Double Column Ties: These are foundational ties used to secure the wrists, ankles, or other body parts. They form the basis for more complex ties.

Square Knot: A simple knot used to connect two pieces of rope securely.

Half Hitch: Useful for starting and finishing ties, creating a stable foundation for more complex patterns.

Friction Knots: These knots, such as the Munter Hitch, are used to control the tension in the ropes.

Tying and Binding Techniques

TK (Takate Kote): Also known as the box tie, this tie is commonly used to restrain the arms. It forms a visually striking pattern on the chest.

Karada: A full-body tie that wraps around the torso, creating intricate patterns. It is both decorative and functional.

Ebi (Shrimp) Tie: A hogtie variation that restricts movement by binding the wrists to the ankles behind the back.

Exploring Shibari Ropes and Ties

Hemp vs. Silk vs. Nylon: Choosing the Right Rope:

Hemp:

Pros: Hemp ropes are popular for their natural feel, flexibility, and grip. They soften over time with use, molding to the body.

Cons: They can be abrasive on the skin, and some people may have allergies to hemp. It requires a breaking-in period to become more pliable.

Silk:

Pros: Silk ropes are smooth, luxurious, and have a sensual feel against the skin. They are less likely to cause friction burns.

Cons: They can be more slippery than other materials, making intricate ties more challenging. They are also less durable than hemp or nylon.

Nylon:

Pros: Nylon ropes are smooth, strong, and less likely to cause allergies. They are also readily available and easy to clean.

Cons: They can be less forgiving and have less grip compared to natural fibers. Some find them less aesthetically pleasing.

CHAPTER THREE
Types of Knots: From Basic to Advanced

Single Column Tie: Used to secure one limb, such as a wrist or ankle.

Double Column Tie: Used to secure two limbs together.

Square Knot: A basic knot used to connect two ropes securely.

Bowline Knot: Creates a non-collapsible loop, often used in Shibari for specific ties.

Munter Hitch: A friction knot useful for controlling tension in the ropes.

Somerville Bowline: A more complex knot that forms a secure loop.

Creating Secure and Comfortable Ties:

Even Pressure Distribution: Ensure that the pressure from the ropes is evenly distributed to avoid discomfort or injury.

Checking Circulation: Regularly check the tied person's extremities for signs of numbness, tingling, or discoloration, which could indicate circulation issues.

Safe Words: Establish clear communication and use safe words to ensure the person being tied can communicate any discomfort or concerns.

Experimenting with Different Rope Textures and Thicknesses:

Texture: Different ropes offer varying textures, from smooth to more textured. Experiment to find what feels most comfortable for both the person being tied and the one doing the tying.

Thickness: Thicker ropes may distribute pressure more evenly, but they can be less versatile. Thinner ropes allow for more intricate ties but may create more focused pressure.

Remember that personal preference plays a significant role in choosing ropes and ties. It's often a good idea to try out different materials, knots, and techniques to discover what works best for you and your partner.

Foundational Shibari Patterns

Here are brief descriptions of the foundational Shibari patterns:

Hanemaki: The Fundamental Shibari Tie:

The Hanemaki is a basic and versatile tie often used as a starting point in Shibari. It involves wrapping the rope around the torso in a way that creates a secure and decorative binding. The tie can be adapted for various purposes, including chest harnesses and full-body bindings.

Ashigarami: Binding the Legs:

Ashigarami focuses on binding the legs and is an essential tie in Shibari. It can be used to create leg harnesses, tie the ankles together, or secure the legs in a specific position. This tie can be integrated into more complex patterns or used independently based on the desired outcome.

Tatemaki: Binding the Arms:

Tatemaki is a tie that involves binding the arms, creating either a decorative arm harness or securing the arms in a specific position. This tie is often used in combination with other patterns to enhance the overall aesthetic and functionality of the Shibari scene.

Nukigake: A Basic Suspension Technique:

Nukigake is a fundamental suspension technique in Shibari. It involves lifting the tied person off the ground using the ropes in a controlled and safe manner. Safety is of utmost importance when practicing suspensions, and it requires advanced knowledge of anatomy, weight distribution, and proper knotting techniques.

It's essential to approach Shibari with caution, especially when attempting suspension techniques, as they involve a higher level of risk and require advanced skills. Beginners should focus on mastering foundational ties and patterns before attempting more advanced and potentially risky techniques.

Before engaging in Shibari, it is strongly recommended to seek education from experienced practitioners, attend workshops, and prioritize safety.

Single Column Tie: This is a foundational knot used to secure a single limb or body part. Various versions, such as the Somerville Bowline, offer different aesthetics and levels of security.

Double Column Tie: Involves tying two columns (usually two limbs) together. This can be done symmetrically or asymmetrically, providing different sensations and visual appeal.

Diamond Pattern (Takate Kote): This intricate pattern involves multiple wraps and crossings, creating a diamond-shaped configuration on the torso. It is often used in upper-body ties.

Karada: A full-body tie that involves creating a series of intricate patterns around the torso, often emphasizing the breasts and genital area.

Futomomo (Leg Tie): Involves tying the thighs together, creating a decorative and restrictive binding.

CHAPTER FOUR
Suspension Techniques and Equipment

Single-Point Suspension: Involves lifting the tied person by a single point on the body, typically a chest harness. Safety considerations, including weight distribution and the use of a load-bearing point, are crucial.

TK (Takate Kote) Suspension: This involves using the diamond pattern discussed earlier as a foundation for a safe and secure full-body suspension.

Suspension Lines: High-quality and load-tested ropes specifically designed for suspension play are essential. Carabiners, suspension rings, and other hardware are used to connect the ropes to a suspension point.

Safety Measures: Prioritize safety by understanding weight limits, regularly inspecting equipment, and having emergency procedures in place. Always have a spotter present during suspensions.

Exploring Sensuality and Intimacy:

Feathering: Lightly dragging fingertips or soft materials across the skin while bound can enhance sensory pleasure.

Communication: Maintain open and honest communication throughout the experience. Check in with your partner regularly and establish safe words or signals.

Mindfulness: Encourage a mindful approach to the experience, focusing on the sensations, emotions, and connection between partners.

Temperature Play: Integrate warm or cool sensations using props like warmed oils or ice cubes to enhance the sensory experience.

Ethical Considerations and Safe Practice

Consent: Ensure that all parties involved provide informed and enthusiastic consent. Discuss boundaries, limits, and expectations before engaging in Shibari.

Communication: Establish clear communication channels between partners. Use non-verbal cues, check-ins, and a safe word system to maintain ongoing consent.

Continuous Learning: Stay informed about new techniques, safety protocols, and best practices. Attend workshops, read books, or seek guidance from experienced practitioners.

Privacy and Discretion: Respect the privacy of those involved and be discreet about your Shibari activities. Not everyone may be comfortable with the public disclosure of their involvement in BDSM practices.

Aftercare: After a session, provide emotional and physical support through aftercare. This may include comforting, hydrating, and maintaining a reassuring presence for your partner.

Engaging in Shibari or any form of bondage requires careful attention to safety to ensure the well-being of all participants. Here's a general safety guide and some emergency procedures to consider:

Safety Guide:

Communication:

Establish clear communication between partners before starting any Shibari session. Discuss boundaries, expectations, and any potential concerns.

Establish a safe word or gesture that allows the person being tied to communicate discomfort or the need to stop the activity.

Education:

Learn proper Shibari techniques from reliable sources. Attend workshops, read instructional materials, or seek guidance from experienced practitioners.

Understand the anatomy, including nerve locations and areas to avoid tying too tightly.

Consent:

Ensure that all participants provide informed and enthusiastic consent before engaging in Shibari.

Regularly check in with each other during the session to ensure ongoing comfort and consent.

Materials:

Use high-quality, non-abrasive ropes designed for Shibari to minimize the risk of injury.

Regularly inspect and maintain your ropes to ensure they are in good condition and free from defects.

Avoiding High-Risk Areas:

Be cautious around joints, major arteries, and nerve clusters. Avoid tying directly over the spine or on joints in ways that could cause injury.

Release Mechanisms:

Have quick-release mechanisms readily available, such as safety shears or scissors, to cut the ropes in case of an emergency.

Observation:

Continuously monitor the person being tied for any signs of discomfort, numbness, tingling, or discoloration.

Be aware of circulation and breathing. If there are any concerns, release the tie immediately.

Environment:

Ensure the play area is free of hazards, and there's enough space for movement.

Keep emergency equipment (first aid kit, phone, etc.) within reach.

Emergency Procedures:

Communication Breakdown:

If a safe word or gesture is used, immediately stop the activity and assess the situation.

If communication breaks down, have a predetermined signal to stop the activity.

Nerve or Circulation Issues:

If the person being tied experiences numbness, tingling, or discoloration, release the tie immediately.

Check for any signs of injury and provide first aid as necessary.

Breathing Difficulties:

If there are any signs of respiratory distress, release the person from the tie immediately.

If needed, perform CPR and call for emergency medical assistance.

Equipment Failure:

In the event of equipment failure, such as a rope becoming too tight or a knot becoming inaccessible, have safety shears or scissors nearby to cut the ropes quickly.

Discomfort or Panic:

If the person being tied expresses discomfort or panic, release the tie immediately.

Provide emotional support and assess for any physical distress.

Thank you for purchasing "Shibari for Beginners"!

We want to express our heartfelt gratitude for choosing "Shibari for Beginners" as your guide into the captivating world of Shibari. Your purchase not only supports our work but also signifies your curiosity and openness to exploring new aspects of intimacy and connection.

This book is carefully crafted to provide you with a comprehensive introduction to the art of Shibari, offering step-by-step instructions, beautiful illustrations, and insights into the rich history and philosophy behind this ancient Japanese practice.

As you embark on this journey, we encourage you to approach Shibari with respect, communication, and a sense of adventure. Whether you are a complete beginner or have some experience, the techniques and principles shared in this book are designed to enhance your understanding and enjoyment of Shibari.

Please feel free to reach out to us if you have any questions or if there's anything specific you'd like to explore further. Your feedback is invaluable to us as we strive to create content that enriches and educates.

Once again, thank you for choosing "Shibari for Beginners." May your exploration into the art of Shibari bring you not only new skills but also a deeper connection with your partner and a heightened sense of intimacy.

Wishing you a fulfilling and enjoyable journey,

THE END